Transcend
Your Diagnosis

Transcend
Your Diagnosis

Mapping a Path to Optimal Well-Being

BY CINDY PAINE
WITH MARGARET BROWN

ISBN: 978-0-578-60998-0

Book Design by Jane Perini, Thunder Mountain Design
First Printing, 2020
OWB Publications
Palm Beach Gardens, FL

www.cindypaine.com

DISCLAIMER

This book tells my story—my choices. The choices
I made on my journey to becoming cancer-free may not suit
everyone. While my wish is to help others transcend and
thrive beyond cancer or any challenge they may
face, nothing in this book constitutes or replaces
professional medical advice.

No suggestions or practices outlined in this book
should be considered as medical advice. Each individual
diagnosed with cancer or any other ailment should seek
competent medical advice, and follow any treatment option
they deem suitable for their individual circumstances.

This book is not intended to be and does not present itself
as a substitute for professional medical advice.

Table of Contents

Note to the Reader

Dear Reader,

In this book I will be sharing my own story to inspire
and empower you. Consider the possibility that the
diagnosis, challenge, or unexpected experience you
are facing is a catalyst in your life. As you read this
book, take time to reflect on your own challenge
when you do the Personal Well-Being Practices.

Through clearing my own fears and limiting beliefs
around my diagnosis, and then connecting to my
innate power and inner wisdom, I have been able
to create Optimal Well-Being for myself. This life-
affirming path of Optimal Well-Being was a gift I was
given in the face of my cancer during a meditation.

I now know this gift was not only for me. It was
given to me to share with the world. We are spiritual
beings having a human experience. We are more
powerful and imbued with attributes to overcome
any challenge than we have been led to believe. I
have taken my cancer diagnosis and used it to uplift,
inspire, and transcend. I have laid out a path that has

worked for me to achieve that goal. I invite you dear readers to step onto and walk this path. Transcend your diagnosis and create Optimal Well-Being, now!

I am blessed with the support of Nandini Gosine-Mayrhoo, our brilliant editor; Gurunam Kaur Khalsa who reviewed the book; Jane Perini's beautiful artistry for our cover and layout; and Jean-Noel Bassior who shepherded us through this process as our book coach. I couldn't have written this book without my writing partner, Margaret Brown, who continues to act as the organized left brain to my creative right brain. Thank you also for the ongoing loving support of my friends and family.

Blessings of love and light,
Cindy Paine

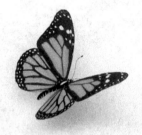

What the caterpillar calls
the end of the world,
the master calls a butterfly.

~ RICHARD BACH

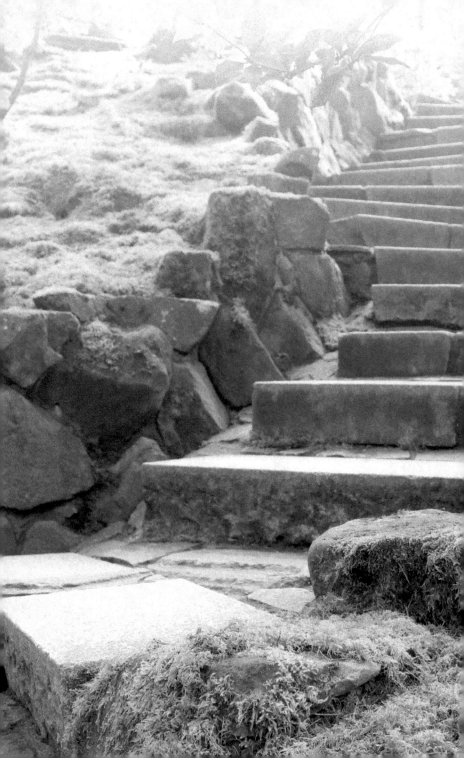

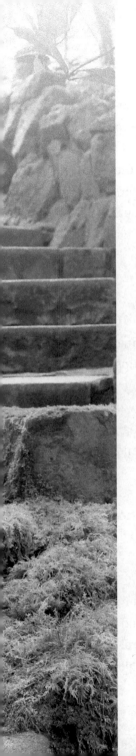

Introduction

Is this book for you?

I had cancer.

While this book is a re-telling of
my experience with cancer, I feel
anyone with any kind of diagnosis
from diabetes to MS could benefit
from this book and reading about
my journey.

I share insights and tools that can
help you transcend any challenge—
the sudden death of a loved one,
dealing with addiction, divorce, or
any experience where the choice is
either to respond as a victim or be
VICTORIOUS!

Take your biggest challenge and
apply the method to your situation.
When I was diagnosed I had two
choices... be a victim, full of
fear, paralyzed by the future... or

walk my talk as a student and teacher of self-love, empowerment, and manifestation. An unexpected message of divine inspiration led me to choose to be a powerful co-creator of my life and walk the path of Optimal Well-Being in the face of my cancer. This is the message that I'm here to share with you.

Big challenges present us with big choices.

What if life is different than what we thought and what we were taught? What if there is more to life than graduating school, finding a job, finding our perfect mate, maintaining good relationships, and getting money? What if life is really about growing and rising above our circumstances? And what if those circumstances are the vehicles through which we can really discover what is important and uncover who we really are?

Everyone always talks about "surviving cancer." I didn't just want to survive cancer, I wanted to THRIVE and surpass all expectations!

If we really are spiritual beings having a human experience, is it possible that challenges and circumstances that seem beyond our control occur to give us the opportunity to step into our power and transcend these challenges?

I chose to triumph over the negative and find that power within to climb up and over any limitations the disease might have given me physically, mentally, emotionally and spiritually. I stepped on my path of Optimal Well-Being... I can tell you, I have found my greatest Self!

CHAPTER ONE

Diagnosis

*Life's challenges are not supposed to paralyze you,
they're supposed to help you discover who you are.*

~ BERNICE JOHNSON REAGON

I have always been a very healthy person and my role model was my grandfather, who lived to be 103 years old. I felt I could easily attain that. There had been no cancer in my family until my father was diagnosed and passed away from melanoma. I always thought this was just because he lived in Florida for many years, was a golfer, and rarely used sunscreen or a hat. I guess I just chalked up his cancer as an anomaly.

One day while making love with my boyfriend Carl, he discovered something on my breast that felt like a lump. He and I had a trip planned to visit a friend in Michigan that weekend. For the entirety of that trip,

I was in my head, fearful of what this lump on my breast meant, wondering if it was cancer. The word *cancercancercancercancercancer* was running through my head. Even though I knew I had scheduled my doctor's appointment for the following Monday, I could hardly be present with friends the whole weekend.

I went to see the doctor, he did a biopsy, and he assured me that he felt it was a cyst which calmed my nerves. He even prescribed something for the cyst which I was to pick up at the pharmacy.

While at the pharmacy counter, for some reason the prescription was not there. This gave me pause, and I felt a low rumble in the pit of my stomach. My brain said, it's nothing, they just forgot to call the pharmacy. As the pharmacist was calling the doctor's office, that low rumble began to intensify. My heart beat faster. My brain started screaming *cancercancercancercancercancer* again. The pharmacist told me, "Your doctor wants you to go home and call their office." At this point, everything started moving in slow motion. I had put my prescription glasses on the counter, while I was waiting, but now they were nowhere to be found (and they never were). I was fumbling through my purse and wandering around the store like I was in a bad dream. I now knew the meaning of the words, 'not being in your body.'

I walked the two blocks to my apartment but have
no recollection of that trip. The elevator to the 27th
floor seemed like it took forever. When I called the
doctor, he said, the biopsy came back and YOU HAVE
BREAST CANCER. For me, the words, YOU HAVE
CANCER, sounded like a death sentence. So many
thoughts and fears flooded into my head. It was just
the most terrifying thing I had ever experienced.

My mouth went dry. I almost dropped the phone and
felt faint, I had to sit down. He told me to get in a
cab and get myself to his office immediately, which
scared me even more. I have no memory of leaving
my apartment and traveling to his office. I don't
remember how I got in the cab, paid for it, and found
a seat in the waiting room. The roar in my ears was
deafening.

It felt like I waited for an hour before I sat down with
Dr. Shapiro. He explained the findings of the biopsy
and scheduled me for surgery to remove the lump
the following week. I had so many questions but I
couldn't even speak. He continued to explain, that
until they operated, they would not know whether
the cancer had spread to my lymph nodes. If it
had spread to the lymph nodes, it may require me
to have a mastectomy. That was a rough moment.
I was freaking out! The terror of thinking of no

longer having my breast was overwhelming. I was completely in shock and fear. I now had to live in the unknown until I had the surgery. To this day, when I share this story, it is hard to relive.

It wasn't the surgery that I was afraid of as much as fearing that they would find all this cancer and I would wake up without my breast. I felt like my body had betrayed me. How could I not know that cancer had invaded my body? Talk about feeling like a victim! I felt helpless that my body was forming these cells over which I had no control. I had difficulty sleeping over the next week, but whenever I woke after a night of tossing and turning, the first thought that entered my mind was YOU HAVE CANCER.

Because of lack of sleep, I felt like I was walking around in a stupor. But I still had to function in the world. I had corporate events to attend to in my catering business. I had clients who I was coaching to be powerful in their lives. I had my boyfriend who was looking at me with sad eyes. I had family members calling with fear in their voices. I was in a war with my mind, and at some point during the week I realized I had to snap out of it and make a change in how I was handling this.

Suggested Personal Well-Being Practices

✦

Write out your diagnosis story, allowing
yourself to feel the feelings.

✦

Take a walk and practice feeling those feelings in your
body and send them down into the earth.

✦

Experience the Grounding Meditation at
http://optimalcancerjourney.com/sample-lesson/

CHAPTER TWO

Surgery

*Surround yourself with only people
who are going to lift you higher.*

~ OPRAH WINFREY

When I was scheduled for surgery I reached out to friends and family to let them know. I started getting calls from my loved ones and they all sounded very concerned. Being in the throes of my own fear, I was hyper sensitive to the feelings of others as if they were being blasted from a loud speaker. The one call that had the most impact on me was from my niece Liza. We had always been very close. I could literally feel the fear that was in her voice. She was trying to sound upbeat, but she sounded so scared, I could feel my own fear rising. I didn't want to be affected by the fears of others. I wasn't sure where this came from, but out of my mouth I said, "I realize that you are scared, but here's how it's going to go... the surgery is going to be great, they are going to find that the tumor is small and encapsulated, the lymph nodes won't be affected, and the cancer will be gone." And then I told her, "I love you Liza, and if you can hold this vision with me, great! Otherwise, right now, I need to be surrounded with people who can steadfastly hold my vision." She agreed, and I continued to share that vision with all the people around me.

Even before switching professions and becoming a coach full-time, I was always a student of personal growth. One of the tools I studied and used quite often was Visioning. Visioning is writing a story about what you want to have happen in the best case scenario, picturing the perfect outcome. In my conversation with Liza I had the realization that I have this tool, I can write a vision for my surgery. At least that was something I knew I could do for myself. I could focus my thoughts on the vision instead of the *cancercancercancercancercancer* mantra that was playing in my head. I continued to flesh out my vision. Wrote it down and shared it with my people. This was my vision:

I wake up the day of surgery confident of a good outcome. I go to the hospital, calm and ready.

Everyone from the moment I enter the hospital—
support staff, nurses, attendees, the anesthesiologist
and the surgeon—is warm and welcoming. I see
them all well-rested and ready to perform a great
surgery. The surgery goes well and they do the
best job they have ever done. They get all the
cancer. It is encapsulated (fully enclosed) with no
lymph node involvement. It is non-aggressive, slow
growing, stage one. The best possible news! I wake
up after the surgery and I am cancer-free, forever!
I have a quick recovery so I can fully return to my
wonderful life.

After writing this vision I remembered something I
learned from Dr. Wayne Dyer, one of my inspirational
teachers. He would always suggest reading your
vision before going to sleep at night so it can marinate
in your subconscious without the "yes buts" that get in
the way. So that's what I did.

I not only read it at night, but read it several times
a day. Every time the fear would creep into my
consciousness I would change my thoughts and read
that vision. My new vision was what I now shared
with all my loved ones. This vision gave them hope
also, and seemed to totally shift the tone of our
conversations.

On the day of the surgery I went to the hospital and was warmly greeted by everyone just like I had written. I remember the nurse giving me something that made feel peaceful and put me on a magic carpet ride to happy-land. I was relaxed. The next thing I remember was coming out of surgery and my surgeon was there smiling. He told me I was one of the lucky ones. The cancer was the size of a nickel. It was encapsulated. No lymph node involvement. It looked like it was slow growing. Exactly as my vision was written!

Suggested Personal Well-Being Practices

✦

Create a vision for where you are on your diagnosis journey. Write about your desired outcome.

✦

Practice reading it before you go to sleep at night and feel the feelings of having achieved it.

CHAPTER THREE

Post-Surgery

You, yourself, as much as anybody in the entire Universe, deserve your love and affection.

~ BUDDHA

When I arrived home after my surgery I laid down on the couch for a while and rested. Carl was with me and I realized I was still very tired. After a few hours of watching TV, I looked up and it was five o'clock. Like I had done every other day at five, I robotically got up to cook dinner. Unbeknownst to me the anesthesia that I had been under was affecting me badly. I started to feel dizzy and the room began to spin. I dropped to the floor and fainted. Carl had difficulty waking me up, so he called 911.

As my eyes began to open, I remember seeing two strangers hovering above me. The ambulance drivers were a young man and woman. They began checking my vitals and asking me questions. The young man asked me what I was doing at the time that I fainted. I said I had just gotten up to make dinner. The woman paramedic had very kind eyes, and just looked at me with a smile. She said the probable reason I had fainted was the anesthesia, which affects everyone differently, but can make some people very dizzy. It is recommended that after any surgery one really needs to rest because your body has undergone a trauma.

She had a twinkle in her eye and quietly said to me, "We women always feel like we have to take care of everyone around us. It is just how we are trained. Maybe you can let him cook the dinner tonight, and you take care of you." This was a big "aha" moment for me. I realized then, that even after undergoing cancer surgery, I thought it was my duty to make dinner that same day. I was definitely brought up to serve, and this was another example of sacrificing myself to serve another. Self-care was not in my vocabulary at that time.

The paramedics said goodbye and I sat Carl down and had a talk with him about the idea of having him take over some of the household duties. He was more than happy to do that, and he was a much better cook than I. This was a great lesson, albeit somewhat dramatic having to call 911, to begin my journey of asking for help and letting others give to me.

Since I have been working with cancer survivors, I have noticed that many people who get cancer are not the best at allowing others to take care of them. A nurse friend of mine, once shared with me that breast cancer patients are often like mothers literally breast-feeding the world, and themselves last. I realized that I came into this life as a caretaker, taking care of everyone else before myself. It was as if this was part of my soul. This experience with the paramedics was a lesson I needed to learn in order to heal, to undo my training as a caretaker. This was the beginning of my journey of loving myself and realizing that it is not selfish but SACRED!

From this point on I became a student of self-love. The notion of self-love is not selfish. Numerous people I talk to tell me that they were told growing up that working on their self is indulgent, egotistical, and narcissistic. Women in our society, especially, are taught to care for and focus on everybody else and not think about themselves. Men, generally, also do not take the time to look after themselves; they make work and productivity their priorities. Societal conditioning does not naturally lead us to look inward to self-reflection. Sometimes it takes a "leveling" like

a devastating challenge or health diagnosis before
we will allow ourselves to pause. Loving ourselves,
making ourselves a priority, working on ourselves, and
clearing our issues incorporate the most unselfish,
sacred act we can do in a lifetime. It is imperative
that we shift from believing that our personal work is
selfish to knowing our personal work is sacred.

It is easy to forget that we are here on this planet to
create, enjoy, and celebrate! One of the first things
I did as a student of self-love was to ask myself,
"What makes me happy?" I put all of those things in
a list and then prescribed for myself a Daily Dose of
Happy! Here are some of the things that are on my
list and may be on your list also:

✦ Petting and playing with animals
✦ Music
✦ Cooking
✦ Talking or going out with my girlfriends
✦ Seeing an uplifting movie
✦ Reading something inspiring
✦ Working in the garden
✦ Dancing with abandon
✦ Eating a great meal
✦ Singing
✦ Exercising
✦ Taking a nice walk or bike ride

✦ Seeing a sunset
✦ Being in nature
✦ Taking a bubble bath with candles
✦ Making love
✦ Acting like a kid, eating ice cream
✦ Intimate connections
✦ Playing with children
✦ Connecting with an old friend
✦ Learning something new
✦ Playing an instrument
✦ Going to a concert or museum
✦ Flying a kite
✦ Going to a beach

Suggested Personal Well-Being Practices

✦

Write about a time when you put another first
at the expense of yourself.

✦

Make your own list of self-loving practices
you can do daily.

CHAPTER FOUR

The Plan

You get in life what you have the courage to ask for.

~ OPRAH WINFREY

After surgery, my next step was to make an appointment with my oncologist. I showed up for my appointment with the Chief Oncologist of St. Joseph's Hospital, Chicago. His office was on the top floor of the hospital. The office was huge with beautiful views of Lake Michigan. His desk was practically the size of my bed. I fixated on one wall which displayed his diplomas and certificates. There were so many! I was impressed.

Dr. Meyer (not his real name) greeted me. He was tall, over six feet, an attractive man in his 40s. He was friendly and warm. We sat down and he began by going over the findings from my surgery. He reiterated what the surgeon had told me: it was a slow growing cancer; it was encapsulated, it was stage one and there were no lymph nodes affected which means the cancer hadn't traveled to other organs. He said that the type of cancer I had was the type you might see in an 80 year old, very slow growing. This was all good.

Then Dr. Meyer went into a conversation about preventing the cancer from coming back. He suggested radiation treatments for 60 days. The radiation would be concentrated on the area from where the tumor had been removed, and would just take a few minutes daily. I had heard stories of people developing burns, but he assured me that because of the location and type of cancer, I wouldn't experience that. He also suggested the drug Tamoxifen and explained that it is a pill taken twice a day usually for approximately three to five years. I wasn't thrilled with this but I was expecting it. At the time, Tamoxifen was a relatively new drug and the reports were promising to prevent re-occurrence. I was open to whatever would make this cancer go away and not come back.

What happened next stopped me in my tracks. He told me I would be receiving chemotherapy. He brought out charts and graphs explaining that there was a four percentage point advantage if I took chemotherapy. Chemotherapy at this time wasn't what it is today. It was, and still is, a cocktail of drugs which targets cells that grow and divide quickly, as cancer cells do. Unlike radiation or surgery, which target specific areas, chemo works throughout your body and can also affect some fast-growing healthy cells, like those of the skin, hair, intestines, and bone marrow. That's what causes some of the side effects from the treatment. Of course, I know this now, but at the time I was just going on what I knew about chemo, that the patient can get very, very sick. This just didn't add up for me. With everything he had said before about the type of cancer I had, it just didn't seem necessary to do chemotherapy. I wanted to build up my immune system, not tear it down. For me, I felt the greatest defense would be a strong immune system.

My intuition was screaming *nonononononono* to the chemotherapy!

As I started to protest the chemotherapy plan, things started to get heated. Dr. Meyer referred back to his charts and graphs, continued to explain best and worst case scenarios. It all seemed so full of fear and dire consequences. I almost got the feeling that I was at a car dealership and I was being 'sold' chemotherapy. The more he talked, the more I felt solid in my resolve.

And let me say here, that I realize that this path is not for everyone. In some cases, chemotherapy is definitely required. And I'm not someone who doesn't believe in modern medicine. I had been brought up to believe what a doctor tells you, and to respect authority. Who do I think I am anyway? I was in a lot of mental conflict. But there was this other part of my being that was very clear. This was not the path I was going to take. I found myself standing up, all 5'2" of me, and telling this big man with all the power, in his impressive office in the sky, "Thank you very much, Dr. Meyer. I am happy to take your other suggestions, but I will not be doing chemotherapy." And I walked out of his office.

Later that day I got a phone call from my internist and she said that Dr. Meyer had immediately called both her and the surgeon, telling them that they needed to compel me to do the chemotherapy. They both looked at the data and supported me in my decision. Of course, there were no guarantees, but they both agreed that chemotherapy was not necessary in my case.

This was an extraordinary moment for me. Up until that time there weren't many times in my life where I stood up to authority. There was a growing power inside of me. My intuition was stronger. I had the ability to trust my sense of knowing and follow my heart. It was empowering!

Suggested Personal Well-Being Practices

✦

Make a list of times you followed your intuition and it worked.

✦

Make a list of the people and places where you are not speaking up in your life.

CHAPTER FIVE

Optimal Well-Being

Intuition is a spiritual faculty that does not explain,
but simply points the way.

~ FLORENCE SCOVEL SHINN

The next few weeks were a whirlwind. Every morning I would get up, take my Tamoxifen, and get ready and go to the hospital for my radiation treatment. My emotions were up and down, varying from optimistic to melancholy. I was angry that I had to think about cancer. I was fearful of re-occurrence. I was mad that this cancer occupied so much of my awareness. I just wanted to get back to my life before this "intruder" showed up and took over. While having a bitch session with one of my friends, she reminded me that I used to mediate and it always seemed to make me more peaceful. I had to admit that I had gotten pretty

removed from my "conscious self." Just like many
people, my self-care ebbed and flowed through my
day-to-day life. I couldn't really imagine at this
time in my life my mind being quiet enough to
meditate again. I surrendered, sat down and went
into meditation. It took a few weeks for my mind to
be quiet enough for the meditation to be of value.
But I committed to it and was going to continue even
though I wasn't really enjoying it. With this practice
I also picked up my journal, just writing my thoughts
and feelings, to help me come back to myself.

One Sunday morning I got up early before the sun
came up and went out to my patio. It was still dark,
quiet in the world and peaceful, the only sounds I
heard were the birds singing as they arose. I decided
to meditate. As I was meditating, many thoughts
went through my mind, and as always, it was difficult
to quiet them. I began to relax and go deeper. I had
a few moments of getting into what people who
meditate call, "the gap." This is the space in between
the thoughts when everything becomes quiet.

I was bathing in this deliciousness when I heard
something, almost like a whisper from within. I
couldn't quite make out the words. I continued to
listen expectantly. The words became louder and
clearer. I even began to see these words as if on a

chalk board in my mind's eye. "Optimal Well-Being."
My first thought was, "What does that mean?" At
that point, I began to come out of my meditation. I
had no idea why these words were coming into my
awareness. While I understood the meaning of the
words, I did not know what they meant to me in the
unfolding of my journey. I felt like my guidance was
trying to get my attention. It was so jarring that I
came out of my meditation and quiet space. I grabbed
my journal and wrote the words "Optimal Well-
Being." Since I didn't know what this meant, I made a
decision to let these words percolate in my mind.

I spent the next few days pondering the meaning
of these words that had inserted themselves into
my consciousness. In my journal I wrote the words,
"What DOES optimal well-being mean, and what
could it mean for me?"

A light bulb went on. I caught my breath. In a
moment, I could see my future laid out before me.
Any remaining fear or trepidation about my cancer
slipped away and I was filled with a surge of power!
I was not only going to survive the cancer, but I
was meant to THRIVE! I understood that to achieve
Optimal Well-Being, I had to become the very best
version of myself physically, emotionally, mentally,
and spiritually. At this point, I wasn't sure how, but

I was up for the task and was committed to begin on that path. The way to accomplish this was to use the tools and techniques that I had created from all of my years of study, the visualizations and exercises that I had been using in my retreats and workshops... I was going to be my own guinea pig using these tools to achieve Optimal Well-Being in the face of cancer. I was going to live! I was going to thrive! And I was going to spread that teaching and healing to the four corners of the world and help everyone else who was afflicted with a frightening medical diagnosis!

And so my Optimal Well-Being journey began!

Suggested Personal Well-Being Practices

✦

Write out what the words "Optimal Well-Being"
could mean for you.

✦

Take some time to quiet your mind: take some slow deep
breaths, meditate or download a relaxation app.

CHAPTER SIX

Physical Well-Being

Believe you can and you're halfway there.

~ THEODORE ROOSEVELT

S o there I was after hearing the words "Optimal Well-Being"... I felt like I had been assigned a divine mission. The first thing that came to me was to define the words optimal well-being for myself in different areas of my life: *physical, emotional, mental* and *spiritual*. The dictionary definition of the word optimal means "most desirable." But to me, and in this context, the word "OPTIMAL" meant to go beyond what I thought was possible.

My definition of Optimal Well-Being could be different from what Optimal Well-Being means to you.

Physical Well-Being. I contemplated what physical optimal well-being might mean for me and began to define it.

- ✦ Endless energy
- ✦ A fit body
- ✦ Vibrancy
- ✦ Healthy Diet
- ✦ Strong immune system
- ✦ Challenge myself athletically
- ✦ Agelessness

Wow! I was somewhat daunted by my own list, but there was a part of me that was excited. Where and how do I begin to create this for myself? I started sharing my goals for my optimal physical self with some friends and one of them who had been through her own challenge with diabetes had been seeing an MD who was also a holistic doctor. She raved about the results she was getting by using some integrative medicine techniques. I was intrigued enough to make an appointment.

I ended up working with Dr. Martha Howard whose whole practice was aimed at building a strong immune system as a defense for any challenging diagnosis. We began with allergy testing. Her belief is that things to which you are allergic require the immune system to work harder. As a result of the testing I immediately gave up coffee, dairy, gluten, corn, and shrimp (I know!). My energy got better! I also went to her for acupuncture and Chinese herbs which eliminated any symptoms I was having from the radiation treatments.

I decided to embark upon a workout program called "Insanity." This program was popular at the time and was considered *extreme*... the very name Insanity denotes that you have to be crazy to try this. I really ended up loving the results.

I don't want to make this sound like any of this was an easy process. Give up coffee?!!! You have GOT to be kidding! I would just pass by the Starbucks on the corner and pause to smell the aromas emanating from the building.

And those early morning workouts of the Insanity Program? I literally *wanted* to die after the first three days.

Once I got past the first week I started enjoying the results. I had a little more energy and week by week my body seemed stronger and more fit. Instead of coffee I found that a couple cups of chai tea in the morning worked just as well and I enjoyed it. Making the dietary changes, although challenging, really weren't that difficult. There were lots of healthy alternatives to milk and cheese. Gluten free options were becoming more prevalent. I started focusing on eating more fruits and vegetables and eventually didn't crave the heavier foods. Aside from the Insanity workout I began riding my bike again and taking wonderful walks in the morning in nature. Drinking eight glasses of water a day, I had always heard was a good idea, but was never something I did regularly. With my new commitment to well-being I decided to take that on as well. It wasn't that hard to drink two glasses before each meal, one when I woke, and before bed.

Every time I wanted to stop for a cup of coffee, or blow off my workout I would hear Dr. Howard's words in my mind, *"A strong immune system is your best defense!"* And I knew, this was the fight of my life and the fight *for* my life. These commitments I was making were bigger than the desires of my rebellious inner child.

Please know, dear reader, none of this was easy. I had been working on myself and had been helping others on making commitments and holding accountability for a long time. I also had the extra motivation that the cancer could grow again in my body and I was doing everything possible to build the strongest immune system that I could. Your journey will be your journey. I cannot tell you that dietary changes and an "insane" workout regime would work for you in your journey to physical Optimal Well-Being. Go with what feels right for you, knowing what you want to achieve. This is your process and you have to do what's right for YOU.

Suggested Personal Well-Being Practices

✦

What would physical Optimal Well-Being be for you?

✦

List the action steps you can take to achieve physical well-being.

CHAPTER SEVEN

Emotional Well-Being

Accept yourself, love yourself, and keep moving forward. If you want to fly, you have to give up what weighs you down.

~ ROY T. BENNETT, *THE LIGHT IN THE HEART*

n looking at emotional well-being for myself and beginning to discern what that meant to me... I had to be honest with myself, I had a lot of stress at that time. As a lifelong student of personal development, I had studied and researched the mind-body connection and I understood the link between our emotions and physical health. When the body is under chronic stress, the process of the immune system to destroy mutating cells becomes inhibited. I truly believe that the stress in my life contributed to my diagnosis.

At this time, I owned an event planning business and was doing my coaching on the side with a desire to be able to do it full-time. While the event planning business had been successful for several years, corporations were doing more event planning in house, and my business was failing. Getting and keeping corporate clients was becoming more challenging and I was earning less. It was starting to be clear to me that this work was no longer my heart's desire. It felt more like a burden and less of a joy. I really felt alive and fulfilled when I was doing my coaching. I remember coming home after events and feeling mentally and physically exhausted!

I was also noticing that I had become a caretaker to some family members and friends. That was my role. I always picked up the phone when people called me for support. I loved being that "go to" person, and had more than a few who relied upon my counsel and nurturing. Unbeknownst to me, this would become my true calling, doing personal and spiritual coaching with people. While I loved being there for people, if I was being honest with myself, in some cases, the calls were draining, especially in my compromised state. It would be some time before I learned how to manage what felt like energy drains.

But the big one was that I was in a 14-year relationship with my partner Carl. Although we loved each other he had the disease of addiction. It was very stressful. I was distracted a lot of the time. There were mood swings and fights, money problems, legal trouble, and fears for the future. Living with an addict was exhausting!

I began to pay closer attention to the possible link between the fear I felt, and my body developing cancer. I also find it interesting that my cancer was found in the breast. For women the breast is the part of the body that represents care-taking, literally being the source of milk for babies. I was care-taking my business, Carl, my friends and some family. I, myself, was nowhere in the equation of my life. I was not making healthy choices for myself. It was the perfect set up for cancer. I had created the ideal environment for it to grow and be fed.

Where could I start with my optimal emotional well-being? I started with cultivating peace where I could.

- ✦ I started taking walks in the morning.
- ✦ I continued my meditation practice.
- ✦ I practiced being very loving in my self-talk.
- ✦ I listened to inspirational teachers.

✦ I surrounded myself with loving friends who supported me.

✦ I began to say "no" and have boundaries.

✦ I did mirror work, which, as the name implies, involves affirming positive statements while looking yourself in the eye in a mirror.

As I was getting stronger doing these practices, the contrast between peace and chaos became much more vivid to me. Coming in from a walk in the park and opening the door to crazy drama seemed to jump out at me in Technicolor. When I got strong enough, I was able to look at my life and consider making the hard decisions. I realized I needed to walk away from toxic relationships and practice self-care in order to actually achieve optimal emotional well-being. This was not easy, and none of it happened overnight, but I began to take the steps that led to me putting myself first. I eventually would leave my relationship, close the event business, follow my true passion—coaching and inspiring others, and move to Florida to surround myself with peace and beauty.

Suggested Personal Well-Being Practices

✦

Discover and list what is causing stress in your life.

✦

Consider and write down the decisions you need to make
to create peace and optimal emotional well-being.

CHAPTER EIGHT

Mental Well-Being

True health begins with your thoughts. Thinking
about comfort, strength, flexibility and youthfulness
attracts those qualities into your life and body. Dwelling
on illness, fear, disease and pain, does just the opposite.
Your work is to notice and change your thoughts and
move them in the direction of health and happiness.

~ DR. CHRISTIANE NORTHRUP

Every morning I woke up very early to get to the hospital for my radiation treatment at 8 AM. As soon as I walked through those sliding glass doors I began to have thoughts about the cancer in my body. Somehow being in the hospital brought up a lot of fear. I questioned whether the radiation would really work and keep the cancer from returning. I worried that there may be burns on

my body from the radiation. I feared that I wasn't taking the right steps to treat my cancer.

As I entered the room where I took the treatment, I
was always greeted by the same radiation technician,
Susan. I got to know her well and she had a calm
demeanor that would usually put me more at ease.
One day I was sharing with Susan the negative
thoughts I was having every morning. I was telling
her that my mind seemed to have its own stories on
how this journey was going to go. The stories I was
telling myself were more like horror stories than
ones with happy endings. Susan listened intently
and then said something I have never forgotten, "You
know, cancer is really more of a mental disease...
the diagnosis can really impact your thoughts in a
powerful way." I ruminated on this. For me the word
cancer had a very "charged" meaning. Just hearing
the word felt like a death sentence. A diagnosis
of any kind like this can put one in 'fight or flight
mode.' Susan went on to say, "Negative thoughts
cause stress which can have a detrimental effect on
your cells and immune system." Could my negative
thoughts and feelings really affect my prognosis? I
wasn't going to leave it to chance. I felt that the very
best thing I could do was to find a way to deal with
the negative stories I was telling myself. As I left
treatment that day, I realized that to achieve optimal

mental well-being it was imperative that I control my negative thoughts.

I went home that day after radiation and just felt like vegging in front of the TV. I needed to escape. It was October and as I was flipping through the channels all I landed on was either horror movies in celebration of Halloween, an old cowboy movie, or cancer stories recognizing Cancer Awareness Month. Ugh! I felt like I couldn't get away from my negative thoughts! I turned off the TV, and closed my eyes to meditate. The light from the TV was still burned in my mind's eye... that's when I had my epiphany!

My mind was like the television and I have a choice on what I want to see and feel. I can choose the channel of the scary thoughts like the bad horror movies, or place my focus on something beautiful and inspiring. Just like the remote control of the TV, I have the power to change the channel in my mind!

A metaphor that clearly illustrates how our minds work is to think about a runaway stage coach sometimes depicted in old-time cowboy movies. (The cowboy movie had obviously made an impression...) The mind is like the wild horses, with its fears, random negative thoughts and gloom and doom pictures. Most of the time those horses run the show, they are in control. We are the stage coach driver whose job it is to take control of the horses. We are not trained to be disciplined about our thinking, our mind takes us wherever it wants to go. In truth, we, like the stage coach driver, can pull the reins and change our thoughts.

So I sat down and made a list of "go to" thoughts that could replace my negative thoughts and fears. I thought of some of the happiest times in my life, like when I was playing with my dog Jezebel as a little girl, being on the beach in Florida with my family, and hiking in the beautiful red rocks of Sedona. When I observed myself feeling fear or telling myself that gloom and doom scenario, I would consciously change the channel to these positive thoughts— positive pictures which affirmed for me love, life and happiness. When I used this technique, which I would eventually call the Remote Control Technique, I immediately had a change of attitude. And honestly, over time, I had less negative thinking about my cancer. I struggled less with my fears. My thoughts moved from worst case scenario to possibility, and at times even peace.

In addition to working with my thoughts, I was aware of the power of affirmations. Affirmations are positive statements spoken out loud and repeated to affect positive results. Around this time I came home from the hospital and went to my shelves of personal growth books and began looking for affirmations that really spoke to me. Certain words always seem to lift my spirits and help me make that transition from fear to peace. I found a few books and started making a list of the most potent affirmations I could find and put them on a card I could carry with me. This came in handy when I was in the waiting room ready to go in for radiation treatments, sitting in my oncologist's office, or getting a mammogram. These are times when my mind could go negative and get into fear, and I felt I couldn't afford my mind to go there.

My favorite affirmation was "Divine health manifests for me and in me now!" This affirmation came from Catherine Ponder who was one of my favorite prosperity teachers. She also wrote the *Dynamic Laws of Healing*. I would say it as soon as I walked through the doors of the hospital, almost like a shield going up around me. I also said it every time I took the Tamoxifen regimen two times a day.

Here are a few other affirmations I used during my journey, and continue to use on my path of Optimal Well-Being. The following affirmations are from Louise Hay, who healed herself from cancer, and was a mentor to me in my self-love work.

✦ I am in perfect health.

✦ Wellness is the natural state of my body.

✦ My mind and body are in perfect balance.

✦ I feel glorious, dynamic energy.

✦ I love every cell in my body.

Suggested Personal Well-Being Practices

✦

Create a "go to" list of positive thoughts and experiences
that immerse you in good feelings.

✦

Practice using the Remote Control Technique
to discipline your mind.

CHAPTER NINE

Spiritual Well-Being

God is bigger than cancer.

~ANONYMOUS

I was brought up in a Jewish household. For many people spirituality is their religion. For most of my life that was true for me as well. My family observed all the traditions. We kept kosher and every Friday night had Sabbath dinners with my mother lighting the candles and saying the prayers. We practiced the rituals, attended synagogue service and had wonderful family gatherings with delicious food. I embraced the warmth and traditions, but I didn't have a strong connection to the religion itself. To me, even now, Judaism is more a moral code of values and a way of life.

It wasn't until I was in my 20s when during a serendipitous visit with friends to the Beechwold

Clinic, that I connected with something larger than myself. The Beechwold Clinic in Columbus, OH is one of the oldest holistic centers in the country. I attended classes there and met many spiritual teachers who introduced me to a whole other realm in approaching spirituality. In those classes I viscerally experienced the power and presence of God and learned how to access Spirit from within. I had experiences of guided visualizations and meditation. I developed a connection with Spirit and learned about and began trusting my intuition. I studied and practiced tools to go within. This is where I found Spirit. Once I had this experience of connecting with something greater than myself, that was everywhere present and within me too, I began my journey of awakening and my realization that I was co-creating my journey.

I had the awareness that God, the Universe, Spirit is energy that exists everywhere, and within me and all of us. It is the source of all creation. It is from that deep place of connection, being grounded and present, that I understood that *I AM* the co-creator of my life. When I connected with Spirit and experienced the oneness, I not only felt the joy, but I could move forward as a powerful co-creator. When I aligned my innate power with the unseen forces of the Universe, I felt I had more impact on my circumstances. This allowed me to create a powerful possibility for my health and well-being. When I was clear about my thoughts, feelings and intentions, I felt I had a tremendous amount of power to make a difference in my life.

It is from this foundation that I approached my spiritual well-being during my cancer journey. Managing all of the emotional and mental spaces, the fear, denial, grief and anger, and then having my epiphany about Optimal Well-Being—I can only describe it as "being drawn into prayer." The past and the future disappeared, faded into the background, as I became present. Things that previously seemed important didn't seem to matter as much. My outer life dimmed, while my inner life blossomed. I felt I was holding hands with the Spirit within me in a very different way. I spent about three months drawing upon the power of Spirit within me, doing everything I could think of to put myself in alignment with Source. These are some of the things I did:

✦ I connected with nature by taking walks in beautiful parks around my neighborhood.
✦ I was in a constant state of prayer.
✦ I practiced uplifting meditations and visualizations.
✦ I called upon my team of angels and guides.

✦ I requested prayer circles to pray for me.
✦ I spent time in quiet contemplation.
✦ I listened to inspiring teachers.
✦ I surrounded myself with positive people.
✦ I stopped watching TV/news.
✦ I stayed in a place of gratitude.

Suggested Personal Well-Being Practices

✦

Write about what gives you a feeling of
connection with Spirit.

✦

Consider what you can do to support yourself
in deepening that connection to Spirit.

CHAPTER TEN

Putting It All Together

*There are only two days in the year that nothing
can be done. One is called yesterday and the other is
called tomorrow. So today is the right day to love,
believe, do and mostly live.*

~ DALAI LAMA

Daily, I began to practice everything to which I had committed physically, emotionally, mentally and spiritually on my path of Optimal Well-Being.

Physically, I had become much more active than I had ever been. I was committed to my daily walks, my Insanity exercise program, biking (for the first time since I was ten), trying to move my body as much as possible. I pulled out a picture of my grandfather, who lived to be 103. When he was asked for the secret of his longevity when interviewed for a newspaper article, his simple answer was, "Just keep moving." I committed to that practice and do so to this day. I maintained consciousness about the foods I ate, making sure they were healthy and whenever possible organic. I only wanted good things in my body to feed my cells.

Emotionally at this point I had let go of my long-term relationship which no longer felt in-line with my commitment to Optimal Well-Being. I actually needed to release several relationships. This was not easy and required a practice of forgiveness and letting go. Ongoing forgiveness of myself and others became a cornerstone of my healing. I had done an inventory of the stresses in my life and one by one, where I could, began to eliminate them. I was making sure I was doing things to support myself like surrounding myself with loving, nurturing friends, engaging in fun activities, listening to inspiring speakers, and creating a life of peace that fed my soul. I continued my practice of the Daily Dose of Happy and kept the commitment to do at least one of the things on my happy list daily. This kept me in joy.

Mentally, I observed my thoughts and words and was dedicated to a practice of changing the negative narration to positive. I limited my exposure to toxic news, people and experiences. The Remote Control was my favorite tool. A practice of gratitude kept my thoughts on what was joyful. As I focused on that, it kept me in a consciousness of peace. As the saying goes, "What you focus on expands." On my walks I would say out loud ten things I was grateful for that morning and there were times when I kept a journal of my gratitude list. Intention was an important part of my mental well-being. With my morning cup of tea, I would intentionally contemplate how I wanted my day to go, and also focus on what I wanted to create. This practice kept me out of the scary thoughts and on to possibility and opportunities.

Spiritually, I had always enjoyed being in nature and I made more time to immerse myself in outdoor activities—something I continue to this day. When I am out hiking, swimming surrounded by the blue sky, serenaded by the birds, walking upon Mother Earth, I feel connected with Spirit. I meditate every morning, spending some part of each day in silence and contemplation. I read and listen to inspiring and uplifting thoughts that awaken my consciousness. I go to the Center of Spiritual Living every Sunday where I am surrounded by like-minded people and feel supported on my path. I am blessed to coach and write and teach these principles which keep me growing and expanding.

I am very aware that this is a unique time in my life where I am single, live alone, am self-employed as a coach with the luxury of working from my home, which affords me extra time to do many of the things that have kept me in Optimal Well-Being. I truly do not feel that in order to achieve Optimal Well-Being one has to do all of the above. It is really just my passion to be absorbed in all of these practices. I feel in my heart if one were to do at least one or two of these practices for themselves, Physically, Emotionally, Mentally and Spiritually, transcending your diagnosis and creating Optimal Well-being can definitely be achieved!

Suggested Personal Well-Being Practices

✦

Identify and write down two practices in each category
to which you can commit.

✦

Begin by doing two of them this week. Continue
incorporating each practice to which you have
committed into your life until they become routine.

CHAPTER ELEVEN

Machu Picchu

Hardships often prepare ordinary people
for an extraordinary destiny.

~ C. S. LEWIS

I was in the middle of my cancer treatment, and even though I had started to "put it all together," I just felt flat. It was the middle of winter in Chicago. The skies were gray, it was cold, slushy and winter seemed like it would never end. The frustration with the daily grind of going to treatment, and the challenges of my life at that time caused me to feel defeated and depressed. I decided that what I needed was some self-nurturing to feel better.

I made an appointment for a little tune-up with a new chiropractor I had heard about. When I arrived she brought me into her office to learn more about me. She asked me, "Where are you with your cancer treatment? What are your intentions for your outcome? What are your intentions for your session today?" I was surprised by her questions but I appreciated her focus on the big picture of my cancer journey. I told her that I was completing radiation, taking Tamoxifen twice a day and working on my physical, emotional, mental and spiritual well-being. My intention was to be cancer-free, healthy, and I shared with her my "aha" moment in regard to my vision to achieve Optimal Well-Being in the face of cancer. My intentions for the session for that day were to release tension, stress and be relaxed and feel more joyful.

I happened to notice a beautiful picture on the wall behind her desk. It was of Machu Picchu. Machu Picchu had always been a place I wanted to visit. I had spent four years studying Peruvian Shamanism in my 40s and we were taught about Machu Picchu and the sacredness of this special place for the shamans and people of Peru. Machu Picchu defies all explanation and logic. It is a magical, mysterious site located 1,280 feet straight up from the river valley below it—as if suspended in air, yet completely hidden from sight. The Shamans of the Inca were the medicine men, or healers of the tribe. As I gazed at this beautiful picture my vision became clear. I wanted to climb

to the top of Machu Picchu, which I had heard is
a very arduous journey. An image of me standing
triumphantly at the top of Machu Picchu formed in
my mind, symbolizing my healing on every level.
I felt it was a potent symbol of me overcoming
my health and physical challenges, releasing my
limiting thoughts and beliefs, and clearing all my
overwhelming fears.

I was excited by these thoughts and raced home to
find my journal from my Peruvian Shaman studies.
I found several pictures of Machu Picchu and picked
one. I also found a picture of myself and glued it to
the top, proudly standing on the peak. Throughout
my journey I used this image as a symbol to keep me
focused on my goals. As I gazed daily at that picture I
would feel the power coursing through my body, the
thrill of achievement, and the strength and power of
my being. When I can do that, I thought... I know that
I have come to the place of triumph!

As I saw myself standing on the top of Machu Picchu
I got the feeling of being connected to my most
powerful Self and Spirit! This was the vision I wanted
to hold close to my heart. It literally represented
my four Optimal Well-Being goals: Physically going
beyond my limits; Emotionally, dealing with my
fears; Mentally quieting my thoughts; and even

Spiritually connecting with the energy of this majestic mountain. This was me transcending my diagnosis! Through logical thinking I had no idea of how I would achieve my Machu Picchu vision. To me it represented defying all reason, and yet achieving my goal—exactly what I was committed to in overcoming my health challenges, defying all odds and creating Optimal Well-Being for myself.

Suggested Personal Well-Being Practices

✦

Write down the specifics of what Optimal Well-Being could be for you. What are your physical, emotional, mental and spiritual goals?

✦

Not everyone wants to climb Machu Picchu. Is there something you have been afraid to try or felt you couldn't achieve? Has there been something that you have been putting on the back-burner for years? Now is the time to stretch beyond your limitations. With this practice, go way beyond what you think is possible to inspire your journey. For you, it might be creating a beautiful garden, crossing the finish line of a marathon, or writing that book that you've been thinking about.

✦

Pick a personal symbol that represents crossing the finish line. Make sure you really stretch beyond what you think is possible for you.

✦

Find pictures that represent you being, doing and having your goals realized.

CHAPTER TWELVE

Vision

Have a vision. It is the ability to see the
invisible. If you can see the invisible,
you can achieve the impossible.

~ SHIVA KHERA

A t this point on my Optimal Well-Being
journey, I had defined the symbol that
represented achieving my health goals. I
had created the picture of myself standing
on top of this great mountain, having climbed to the
top! I even created what I call a Vision Notebook. I
liked this better than the traditional Vision Boards
which were popular at the time. Vision Boards are
pictures that represent your hopes and dreams glued
to a poster board. I put my inspirational pictures
in a notebook which was easy to carry. I brought
my Vision Notebook to the hospital, and would flip

through it during treatment and in my spare time. My pictures represented me being, doing and achieving my Optimal Well-Being goals. I had pictures of myself, not only climbing Machu Picchu, but traveling to Italy, the Greek Islands, Hawaii, and other destinations on my bucket list. I saw myself in a great relationship enjoying life to the fullest; having dinner in exotic places with my handsome man. I pictured myself sitting cross-legged meditating in a beautiful spa in total peace. I cut out pictures of delicious healthy foods. I cut out pictures of people walking, swimming and bike riding, and generally having a great time in life—healthy, at peace, and empowered! Working with a Vision Notebook fed my subconscious positive pictures which reinforced my intention to achieve Optimal Well-Being.

I decided that the next step for me was to write out a vision to literally "Place my order with the Universe." This vision would create a new powerful program of health and well-being in my mind. I know from the research I have done for my coaching that our behaviors are a result of what we observed and recorded in our first seven years of life. Similar to a computer-like program in our mind, the trick is to not necessarily delete the programs that no longer work for us, but to download a louder, stronger program that better serves us. Therefore, creating a vision I could read to myself or out loud was another tool I could use to reinforce my intention and create a new program. As mentioned before, Wayne Dyer recommended reading your vision before you fall asleep each night letting it "marinate" in your subconscious without the "yes-buts." He said that before sleep, most people worry about things in their life, or they have just watched the news, which puts negative, fear based thoughts in your subconscious. This technique of putting what you *want* to create in your subconscious, versus what you don't want to create, is a powerful manifestation tool.

As I sat down to write a vision of Optimal Well-Being I took the goals that I had in each area—physical, emotional, mental and spiritual and wrote them in present tense as if they were occurring now. I used the words "I AM" which invoke the power of Spirit. I addressed all my senses, how it would feel to achieve it, what it would be like, smell like and taste like. I wanted to make the ultimate end result not only feel like it was occurring in the present, but the most important part, is to FEEL the feelings around having already achieved it!

Night after night, week after week, month after month, out loud and with energy, I would read my vision, the last thing I did before I went to sleep,

letting it marinate in my subconscious, believing
without doubt that it would manifest in my life.

How to Write a Powerful Vision

In previous Well-Being Practices, I have suggested
that you get very specific about your intention and
what you want to create. Now I want you to see it.
You should already have some pictures in your mind,
maybe you've even cut out a picture from a magazine
that represents what Optimal Well-Being is to you.
Now, I want you to really tell a story with those
pictures. In Visioning, the mental and emotional
bodies work together to activate our subconscious.
The subconscious is where our minds dwell during
sleep, and is also the vehicle through which our
manifestations come to us. Our subconscious does not
understand what is happening in reality, present time
vs. what is happening in our thoughts or emotions.

As you imagine your creation, the subconscious
will bring you that. The more we can activate our
subconscious to get behind our creation, the quicker
our creation will manifest. The words "I AM" invoke
God, the Universe, your highest self and the universal
flow of energy (or whatever words you want to use to
name your own power). The words "I AM" align you
with Source; it is the presence of Source in action and

invokes the full activity of God. When you say and feel "I AM" you open wide the door to natural flow. When you say "I am not," you shut the door. I always begin my visions with "I AM." At the end of all my visions, I say the phrase, "This or something better, and so it is." This statement opens up the possibilities of even greater manifestations from the Universe, greater than anything your conscious mind may have conceived.

If you can see it, you can believe it. You first have to see it in your mind's eye. You need to create the movie in your mind, and then write it out.

✦ Write your vision as if it is occurring now, in the present tense. Use the word "now" in your vision to pull it into the present, as opposed to something you desire in the future. If you picture your creation occurring in the future, that is where it will stay, it will always be in the future.

✦ Use the words "I AM."

✦ Never write what you do not want. If you write, I do not want cancer in my body, for example, the Universe will give you more of "not wanting cancer." Phrase your visualization naming what you do desire, for example, "I am in Divine, perfect health now!"

✦ Write in as much detail as you can imagine, utilizing all your senses.

✦ As we have said before, the feelings you bring to your visualizations are one of the most important aspects. Get in touch with the joy and the excitement of Optimal Well-Being. Feel what it is like to have it! Turn up the dial of that high joy vibration filling every cell in your body.

✦ At the end of your vision, use the phrases, "For the highest good of all," and "This or something better. And so it is!"

Suggested Personal Well-Being Practices

✦

Write a vision using all the parameters discussed.

✦

Read it each night before you go to sleep,
so it marinates in your subconscious.

CHAPTER THIRTEEN

Forgiveness

You will begin to heal when you let go of past hurts, forgive those who have wronged you, and learn to forgive yourself for your mistakes.

~ ANONYMOUS

One of the cornerstones of my reaching Optimal Well-Being on my cancer journey was forgiveness. In fact, in my work with others, especially on my retreats I often say, "If you only take away one thing from our work together, let it be forgiveness. This alone will transform your life." It certainly has mine!

During my personal growth studies I attended the EST Training created by Werner Erhard. One of the main principles he taught was taking responsibility for everything in your life. EVERYTHING! So where did that leave me with having contracted cancer? If I were to take full responsibility, would it follow that I had in some way caused it? I had the awareness that on some level, I was blaming myself for the things I did or didn't do which caused me to get cancer. I had to consider whether somehow I had created my cancer by staying too long in a toxic relationship, allowing myself to live a very stressful life, eating foods that weren't healthy and all the other things I might have done since birth that I shouldn't have. I obsessed on whether my cancer was a consequence of me having "wasted my best years" spent with an alcoholic and not having the courage to leave that relationship earlier. I wasted a lot of time going over the choices I *should* have made for my Optimal Well-Being *before* I had cancer, wishing for a "do over." Worse yet, how could I be a coach and teacher of all these wellness principles and not even live up to them in my own life? This line of thinking was getting heavier and heavier and causing me to feel bad about myself and my situation. It was time for me to do some work on forgiving myself. If I wouldn't take chemo because it would have harmed my immune system, why would I continue to harbor these toxic thoughts and feelings in my body?

In order to begin a forgiveness practice I began by doing a deep dive into my life and choices. I took

out my journal and asked myself these questions:
With whom was I still angry? What resentments
was I holding onto? Whom have I not forgiven? Are
there things for which I have not forgiven myself?
I listed each incident or person and committed to
doing a forgiveness practice. I answered for myself
why I had stayed in a toxic relationship for so long.
I discovered how I had grown from my stressful
job and enumerated what I learned about myself in
that experience. By hanging on to the shame and
disappointment in myself, I had kept myself in a
place of imbalance and dis-ease and consequently felt
a lack of ease and harmony within my body.

By beginning the practice of forgiving myself
for getting cancer, I realized that what may have
contributed to my dis-ease were ALL of the people
and experiences throughout my life that needed
forgiveness. Even people in my life who had done
things that I felt I couldn't possibly forgive: a brother
who had betrayed me, a girlfriend who slept with
my boyfriend, men who had left abruptly, business
associates who promised things and never followed
through these were some of the many things that life
brings us all, that I was still carrying. As a coach I
hear horrific stories of the seemingly unforgivable! As
I've heard it said, by not forgiving myself or others,
it was like I was swallowing the rat poison, and

expecting the rat to die. When I became completely committed to my own Optimal Well-Being, I knew that I had to let go of the past, stop ingesting the poison and forgive all others, but especially myself.

So now that I had identified the unforgivable, how do I forgive, releasing it once and for all so I wasn't carrying that toxic energy? I realized a long time ago that I had a false belief about forgiveness. Somehow I thought that by forgiving someone I was condoning their bad behavior. That I was somehow saying it was "OK." What I realized, is that by forgiving the person who I felt had transgressed me, I was not condoning the behavior, the act, the words or the hurt. The experience happened. When I choose not to forgive I carry the story. I carry the burden of the anger, outrage, shame and unresolved feelings into my present by continuing to hold onto the past. When I was able to forgive them, I let go of my grudge and all the feelings that were harming me, including the heavy energy of that experience. I was finally free!

With this situation I decided to use some of the tools and techniques I use with my clients. I often suggest the technique of writing to the person that you are angry with or have not forgiven without sending it— saying everything you need to say to feel complete, making sure to get out all the anger and hurt that you may not feel comfortable saying to them in person. This works even if the person is no longer living. I had a long list of people to whom I needed to write. I added a powerful tool of doing a burning ritual I learned studying Shamanism. After writing your letter, you read the letter out loud one last time and burn it with the intention of letting it go.

Another tool I used that was powerful was called the Re-Creation Technique. In this technique you find a good friend and teach them how to hear you without advising or interrupting. My friend Susan and I practice Re-Creation regularly. We have literally been "clearing" our lives for many years. This seems very simple, but when you full out express yourself and someone can really hear you, stuff literally disappears. But the bottom line is that you have to be ready and committed to letting go of the story.

Something I do in my retreats is to have the participants imagine that the person from whom they need forgiveness (or who they need to forgive) is sitting across from them. Then I instruct them to say everything they need to say in order to be complete. This can also be used for yourself by speaking to yourself in the mirror, saying everything you need to say, ending with "I forgive you and love you." Forgiveness is one of the most important keys I used in my journey of Optimal Well-Being! It is an ongoing practice, every day being willing to forgive others, but especially myself.

Suggested Personal Well-Being Practices

✦

Make a list of who and what you have not forgiven.

✦

Try one of the practices such as Writing a Letter and burning it; Re-Creation or Mirror Work.

CHAPTER FOURTEEN

Trust

As you build trust in yourself, your ability
to expand your vision and fully live in your
magnificence is amplified.

~ MIRANDA BARRETT

I mentioned earlier that I had a difficult time trusting my body after I was diagnosed. I felt like my body was betraying me in creating these cancer cells. I just couldn't wrap my mind around it. How did the switch get flipped to start making cancer cells? I had a betrayal of trust with my body.

As babies, we come into the world helpless and open. We need to rely on our parents/family for everything. We trust God, life, family and everyone we are interacting with. It is natural for us to trust. As we grow up we begin to do things for ourselves and not be as dependent upon our family. During life things occur that feel like betrayals. People we believed in said things that we later found out were not true. Situations to which we gave ourselves we later discovered weren't the best for us. When this happens we can begin to put up walls.

In order to heal this, I explored for myself times in my life where I trusted and it didn't work out. Our minds like to hang onto these scenarios, so I had a whole filing cabinet full of times where I felt betrayed. I journaled some of these experiences. I realized I was really beating the drum of that conversation in my mind. I found that because of those experiences and the way I had processed them I was guarded. I have had female coaching clients who have come to me after a failed marriage and told me that they really want to find true love, but they don't trust themselves to pick a good man. They have cut themselves off from wonderful opportunities because of one bad experience.

Now, the flip side of this, of course, is that there are just as many times that I trusted and it DID work out. Our minds like to tuck these scenarios in the back of the filing cabinet. But upon examination I discovered that there were many more times that I trusted and it did work out, than there were when it didn't. I journaled about the times when I listened to that still, small voice within and acted on it. It felt so much better to think of these experiences than the former.

One time in particular comes to mind. I had lived in Chicago for over 25 years. I had built a practice of coaching, led workshops and did speaking engagements. I had a community of like-minded friends that felt like family. My life was comfortable. I had a beautiful apartment in a skyscraper overlooking Lake Michigan and considered Chicago my home. I didn't love the winters, and would sometimes think about moving somewhere warm, but that seemed like something far in the future.

Several circumstances happened all at once that had me thinking about making a change. My apartment was no longer going to be available and I would have to move. I had been working on a book about self-love for about eight years but I was so distracted with my social life and work, I just couldn't get it finished. My sisters and I shared ownership of a beautiful home in Florida, left to us by our parents, which was sitting empty. We weren't sure what we were going to do with the home, we would probably get it ready to sell at some point, but it was available to me. I had an intuition I should go to Florida, live in that home, and finish my book.

Another part of me, the more practical side, put the brakes on! Leave this city that I love—my friends, my work? No way! But this idea just kept coming back and at some point I realized how torn I was about this decision. Am I going to take a leap of faith? I really feel called to finish this book. I'd love to skip a winter here and see what it's like to live in a warm climate. And then there were the "yes, buts": Yes, but what about all my friends? Yes, but what about my practice? What if I can't make it there? And on and on it went.

I reached out to my good friend Terry, to discuss my fears. I laid out my alternatives. All she said was, "Check the evidence, Cindy." The first time she said this, it just annoyed me. What does that even mean? A few weeks later I called her back with a new set of doubts and fears, and she said it again. This time I bit. She explained that having known me for a long time, she knew I had always lived in lovely homes and it had always worked out. So why would I think that this time would be different? She told me to look back at the numerous experiences I had of finding and living in wonderful places. Each time I moved, the places seemed to be getting better and better with each new location.

I did decide to go, but I had a lot of trepidation. Truth be told, I kind of went kicking and screaming. But a small little voice kept pushing me forward. It ended up being a wonderful decision. I was able to oversee the completion of repairs and clean out my parents' home, honoring what they had built. I was able to help my sisters by being there on site to oversee the sale of the house. I found that I loved Florida. It didn't happen overnight but I made new friends that are just as close as my Chicago Tribe.

When we sold the house I was again faced with the need to find a new place. This time, without even calling Terry I applied her "check the evidence" practice when dealing with my fears and doubts about finding my next home. I eventually moved into a house that I adore, overlooking the golf course and water and just as beautiful as any place I've ever lived. I have met new partners in my business, catapulting me to a whole new level of success. The peace and lack of stress where I live now allows me the freedom to constantly create new programs and ways to reach new audiences with my work.

This is a story about trust. It was important in my cancer journey that I trust my body again. I checked the evidence. I reflected on my body's ability to heal. Every time I had a flu, sinus infection, or a torn ligament, my body miraculously always healed itself. I realize cancer is potentially more complicated than what I have had to overcome in the past, but with my faith that everything always has, and still is working out for my good, I chose to believe that this would too.

It was also important for me that I extend this trust to my medical team and the people in my life who I needed to support me during this health challenge. But even more than that, I wanted to trust that God still had a plan for me and that I could trust that something greater was in control. Even though I couldn't see the outcome, I needed to trust that good things would come out of going through cancer.

When have you followed that still small voice inside and it led you to something wonderful? When you focus on these times in your life, you begin to build the muscle of trust which will carry you through the doubts and fears of your cancer journey. Check the evidence. Can you begin to trust that this may all be happening for some greater purpose?

Suggested Personal Well-Being Practices

✦

Write about a time when you have trusted yourself,
or simply trusted the process and things worked out
wonderfully.

✦

Imagine if you were able to trust, what you would
do with your life that you are not currently doing.
Even if you're skeptical, breathe, and allow
yourself to trust the process.

CHAPTER FIFTEEN

Surrender

Try something different. Surrender.

~ RUMI

I can already hear some of you questioning my use of the word "surrender". Why would she be talking about "surrender" in relation to cancer? No way! I'm gonna fight fight fight! You might have decided that in going through this cancer journey, that you were just going to "soldier up" by putting on a strong façade, and in some instances that might be working for you. Most of us try to control our circumstances to survive. In the past I had looked at "surrender" as giving up. I had visions from movies of soldiers in bunkers waving the white flags. The idea of surrendering is scary.

I am using the word "surrender" here to designate *the ultimate form of trusting.* I'm talking about surrender from the perspective of *knowing* beyond a shadow of doubt that the highest good for you is occurring no matter where you are on your cancer journey. Surrender is letting go of control when we get to the place of knowing that *everything* is for our highest good.

I have two very good friends, Eric and Susan, husband and wife, who now live in Sedona. When I met them we all lived in Chicago, this was years before my diagnosis. They are both very adventurous people, but especially Eric. He loves to push himself beyond what he considers his limit. He would do things like ropes courses where you go across mountains on ropes, he would race cars at high speeds, and jump out of airplanes. I kind of looked at him in awe at all of the things he was doing. His wife and I would for the most part stay in our safe little comfort zone and let him be the wild one.

One day, when I was visiting their home, he came home and challenged us both to go to Wisconsin for a full day of training and parachuting. I was so afraid of heights, I balked. There was no way I could imagine myself doing this. He continued to share about how powerful an experience it had been in his life. Susan and I put our heads together and decided to show him! He had thrown down the gauntlet and we took the challenge. I was terrified.

We spent one full day learning everything one needs to know to parachute. Most of the day I wasn't even in my body, I was so scared. I probably didn't even hear half of what the trainer said. But before I knew it, Susan, myself, the instructor and a couple other people were entering a small plane. Was I really going to do this? As a side note, this was a while ago, back then you jumped solo, not like today where you jump in tandem with a seasoned trainer.

So we went up higher and higher. The roar of the plane couldn't drown out the pounding of my pulse in my ears. I remember how small the plane was. It didn't even have a door! It was all wide open and I could see the ground getting farther away. The houses and cars getting smaller and smaller—at one point I thought that it looked like a monopoly set down there. Everything was tiny, tiny, tiny, and I knew that we were very high up in the sky.

The trainer announced that we should get ready to jump and the shortest person goes first. I looked around at the other people. I guess I should say, I looked *up* at the other people, since I was the shortest person on the plane. I had never been so afraid in my life. That's when it hit me, *I was literally going to jump out of this plane!* I had two parachutes on me, but if they didn't open, I was in trouble. I was really facing a life-and-death situation. Even thinking about it today, some 20 years later, it still feels terrifying. My mind told me it was too late to turn back now. I looked at my best friend Susan. I asked, "Is it going to be ok?" I know Susan loves me. She wouldn't want anything bad to happen to me. She told me, "Go for it." I took that trust my friend had in me and my safety into my heart and decided it was okay to go. I stood at that doorway, the wind whipping in my face so hard it was difficult to breathe. We were trained to literally swan dive out into the sky. I took a deep breath and did my swan dive.

I floated out into the air and pulled the cord for my parachute. It opened.

The rest of the time was literally the most incredible experience I had ever had. I was flying through the air. I felt that I flew through my fear of heights. I flew through my anxiety of doing something I was afraid of but did it anyway. My heart was bursting with pride for myself! I began to float down. It was a beautiful fall day in Wisconsin and the trees had turned brilliant colors of orange, gold and red. I was looking down at the canopy of colors and the views were breathtaking. It was an incredible experience of the world being very quiet and peaceful and I was flying!

I eventually landed softly and I was so fulfilled! I had let go and surrendered my fears and I had trusted and it had all turned out wonderfully. I never jumped again, I didn't have to. I had conquered my fears and that experience was enough, I was empowered! From that point on I carried with me pictures that Eric had taken of me during my jump to remind me of that moment of trust and letting go. Every time I would get scared and wanted to control the circumstances I would look at those pictures and remember when I trusted, surrendered, and dove through my fears to have an ecstatic outcome.

Surrendering on the cancer journey was difficult for me to accept. I called upon my parachute experience when I found myself wanting or even believing that I could somehow control every aspect of my cancer journey. While going through the twists and turns that occurred on my journey there were many times I really had to let go. For instance going into the operating room and not knowing what the outcome would be, taking Tamoxifen even though I was against taking an aspirin, doing radiation after considering the possible side effects.

Those were times when I really needed to trust the doctors, trust the treatment and trust God. Surrendering, trusting and letting go to a power greater than myself that wants my good and has my back can create miracles!

Suggested Personal Well-Being Practices

✦

What does Surrender mean to you?

✦

Look at a time in your life when you surrendered, when it felt like you had no control and things worked out.

CHAPTER SIXTEEN

Telling a New Story

If you can't figure out your purpose, figure out
your passion. For your passion will lead you
right into your purpose.

~ BISHOP T. D. JAKES

A t this point on my journey, I had finished my radiation treatments and was taking Tamoxifen. The doctors warned me that I would need to wait for my next breast exam before I should feel like I was out of the woods, but I felt like the coast was clear. I can't really say that cancer ever fully left my consciousness, knowing that I would have to endure regular, and more frequent breast exams, didn't exactly put me at ease.

I decided to go to a support group at the hospital

recommended by my oncologist. Here was a group of women, who had lived through what I was living through, sharing their experiences.

As I listened to each person speak, one repeated theme was women telling their cancer story years after they had been diagnosed. Some of them even seemed like they were wearing that story like a badge—reveling in the telling of their fear and challenges it seemed to be the focus of their lives. I can understand that in the beginning, when you are diagnosed, but years after? The thought crossed my mind, "That's not going to be me. I will not be leading into an introduction of myself with I went through cancer three years ago... five years ago... ten years ago." While I understood that these women were inspiring us with their survival stories, which were so needed within the support group, I wondered about identifying with my cancer journey in such a way.

As a coach I understand the importance of "clearing" your emotions. This means that the emotions are spoken until they are expressed completely and then they are let go. But what I began to notice in my coaching practice was that many people who had had the experience of cancer or any other significant traumatic experience sometimes get stuck in the "story." It appears to be all consuming. I was thinking about this as it related to myself. I teach people, and try to act accordingly, to be aware of the story I tell myself and tell others. When you tell a story you bring the energy of that experience back to yourself. If it's a negative story you might feel down, if it's a positive story you will feel uplifted. Words have energy. What you think and speak out loud you create. By telling this story of illness and identifying with it so completely, they were beating the drum of creating more fear, and certainly not creating Optimal Well-Being. So, for instance, if I am always saying that I am someone who has a hard time being in a relationship, or I never make enough money... I will create more of the same. Telling the cancer story over and over, and identifying yourself as someone who has cancer, is probably one of the worst things we can do. For myself I realized that I needed to create a new story and repeat that new story to create a different outcome.

I spent time thinking about when my cancer was not in my thoughts. What I realized was that when I was fully engaged in my work, at a speaking engagement, coaching clients, or leading a retreat—cancer was nowhere in my thoughts. When my attention was on something other than myself, when I was being fulfilled by my work, when I was having fun with loving friends and family, the thought of cancer was nowhere in my mind. Could that be the key? I remembered a line from a seminar I took where the leader said, "When you have your attention on making a difference and serving others—something bigger than yourself—your issues will disappear."

This was one of the biggest "aha" moments for me on my cancer journey. When I heard the words *Optimal Well-Being* during meditation, that was when I started to look at my cancer journey as a bigger vision. I felt that I had gotten cancer because there was something that I needed to do for people going through cancer. My passion had always been about helping others to achieve their goals and realize how powerful they are. But now that I had gone through cancer, what I was here to do, the reason I'm on the planet, is to use those gifts to help people transcend their diagnosis and achieve Optimal Well-Being. When I keep my focus on others I forget myself. This was something I was experiencing no matter what my mood or situation in my life. When I am working with a client all of the chatter of Self falls away. When I am present, focused, and in service the "little me" is gone and my most empowered Self that knows I can achieve greatness shines forth. For me, I decided to live my life with the passion of my greater purpose, and THIS would be my new story!

At that moment I stepped into my commitment to support others to find their power as co-creators of their experience to achieve *Optimal Well-Being in the Face of Cancer* (the title of my webinar from which this book was adapted).

I encourage you here to begin to put your focus and attention on what you want to achieve. Is there some area in life that you feel passionate about in which you want to make a difference? Begin to journal about something bigger than yourself, something you may have felt was impossible, or too out of reach. Where can your skills, talents and abilities have an impact? How can you change the life of another? This can be something you have been thinking about for a long time, or maybe something that has come up for you recently that you thought you couldn't do because of your life challenge.

Suggested Personal Well-Being Practices

✦

Journal about what may be your goal or higher
purpose for yourself—something you want to achieve
but maybe feels out of reach. What are some action
steps which will take you forward into actually
achieving this Bigger Vision for yourself?

✦

Make a list of your skills, talents and abilities.
Write a new story about your journey.

CHAPTER SEVENTEEN

Mining the Gifts of the Cancer Experience

With everything that has happened to you, you can either feel sorry for yourself or treat what has happened as a gift. Everything is either an opportunity to grow or an obstacle to keep you from growing. You get to choose.

~ WAYNE DYER

I can almost hear some of you thinking, "What? How can I possibly see cancer as a gift?" I know this may be a really hard pill to swallow. I can even say, comparatively, I got off rather easy on my cancer journey. This journey has been much harder on others. Your cancer may have spread, you might have had to endure multiple surgeries, mastectomies, chemotherapy, the list goes on and on. You may be reading this book and be in the middle of your journey, and the pain and the fear are all very present for you. Even considering your cancer as a gift at this point may be impossible for you to conceive. But bear with me, you may find a "diamond in the rough" from this teaching.

With my realization that cancer brought me my life purpose of being able to help people going through cancer, and by holding that as my bigger vision... my heart opened to gratitude. This allowed me to look at cancer through a different lens. A word and practice I use with my clients is "re-contextualizing." What that means is to take an experience and look at the possibility of interpreting it a different way. When you do that, your perception of the actual circumstances begin to shift.

You may have heard a repeated phrase of one of my dearest teachers, Wayne Dyer. He says, "If you change the way you look at things, the things you look at change." I believe this also, and I've seen it work over and over in my own life and in my coaching practice. For example, when you've had a breakup and it's shattering and you really feel the loss, but after time passes, you may eventually get to a place where you possibly ask yourself, "What did I learn from this experience?" Maybe you learned to set boundaries. Maybe you learned to speak up for yourself. Maybe you learned to value yourself more. Many things are garnered from even the worst experiences. So it really does depend on how we look at it. When you change your perception of the events, it feels like the circumstances change, or at least your reaction to those circumstances.

When I sat down to "mine the gifts of my own cancer journey"... (just an aside, I use the word "mine" deliberately because it causes me to picture myself *chipping away at my cancer journey like a miner would,* looking for the treasure)... one of the gifts I received was the awareness of how much of a caretaker I was.

I told the story of how I jumped up to cook dinner even though I had just had surgery. This is a perfect example of caretaking to excess. Taking care of others is a wonderful trait. I came into this life with empathy for others and a need to take care of them. That empathy is what makes me a great coach. What I learned from my cancer journey was that I could no longer take care of others to excess, I also needed to take care of myself. My caretaking had become a "soul wound" having me put others first and myself last, never taking the time I needed to "fill up the tank." A soul wound is a behavior or pattern that you are here to heal. My cancer allowed me the opportunity to hit the pause button on my life and see how I could find balance. This experience also showed me that I was supported by family, friends and loved ones, that I didn't always have to do it all, by myself.

My cancer had me become aware of the stresses in my life and emboldened me to make the changes I needed to make to create a life with less stress. I know that little, or no stress is the best defense against my cancer and supports my immune system to be as strong as possible.

As I have said, I feel very grateful that I am able to contribute to the cancer community. I don't think I ever would have done this fulfilling work if I had not gone through my experience and had my own vision about Optimal Well-Being and proceeded to achieve it.

I definitely feel the preciousness of this life. I am awakened to that experience. My life was more important to me than any unhealthy relationship, than any addiction to food, coffee, or sugar. My physical, mental, emotional and spiritual well-being became number one.

I learned to have more compassion for others. I had always been a strong, healthy person, but sometimes it is only when we have experienced vulnerability ourselves, that we are able to empathize with vulnerability in others. For example, we can never fully understand grief, until we have experienced loss ourselves. While I have always been able to empathize with my clients and their individual circumstances, having cancer myself brought an increased sensitivity and awareness of what it is like to face such a challenge.

I appreciate the people in my life even more. And I am certainly more present, not as much thinking about the past or the future but savoring the now. I have learned to let more love into my life. I have opened myself up more to that possibility and have become more graceful at receiving support.

Challenging things happen in life all the time. Try to look at life as if we are all learning in the classroom. Try to re-contextualize any experience as neither good nor bad, but only as a vehicle through which you learned something. Then, even very challenging experiences become profound. All negatives can become positive. Just like Wayne said, "If you change the way you look at things, the things you look at change." You will then discover your diamonds in the rough.

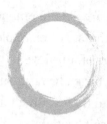

Suggested Personal Well-Being Practices

✦

See if you can uncover what your "soul wound"
could be. A soul wound is a behavior or pattern
that you are here to heal.

✦

Make a list for yourself of the "gifts" you have received
as a result of having gone through your own cancer
experience. These can be things you learned about
yourself, blessings, and/or experiences you have had.

✦

Since "mining the gifts" may be a new practice
for you, continue to look at other challenging
circumstances throughout your life and seek
out the treasures from them.

CHAPTER EIGHTEEN

Unexpected Challenges

*I have always believed, and I still believe, that
whatever good or bad fortune may come our way
we can always give it meaning and transform it
into something of value.*

~ HERMAN HESSE

As of the writing of this book I am approaching my 16th year of being cancer-free and healthier on all levels than ever before.

Physically, I just returned from a trip to Ireland, hiking the Cliffs of Moher. I have reached seven miles (going for ten) on my weekly hikes in Florida. I feel more fit and energetic than I felt in my 20s. I recently took up a new sport called pickleball, similar to tennis, which I play three times a week.

Mentally, I find that what's most powerful for me is to focus on others and something greater than myself. I became very clear this year as I began adapting the *Optimal Well-Being in the Face of Cancer* webinar to a book, that speaking, embracing social media and doing coaching for people going through this journey is the best way I can stay in Optimal Well-Being mentally. Focusing on my purpose to empower and support people to transcend any circumstance keeps me going. When I am doing my work, my concerns and cares disappear.

Emotionally, I am like everyone else, some days I wake up with worries. But I start my day with a meditation, and have recently added yoga to my morning practice. Throughout the day I listen to something uplifting and inspiring and try to focus my thoughts and feelings on what I am grateful for and I always look for the gifts in every experience.

Spiritually, I make a deep connection to nature on my hikes. I go to a Sunday service where I share Spirit with a like-minded community. I belong to a women's circle whose purpose is to uplift and remind us of our divine connection.

I have found the discipline and commitment required to continue doing these things and building on my Optimal Well-Being.

However, there are always challenges. I recently had my yearly mammogram and check-up, which for 16 years had gone perfectly, and that was my expectation. A couple days later I received a call from my doctor saying that I needed to go back for further testing because they thought they had seen something. My original terror when I was diagnosed with cancer returned. I was truly shocked and afraid.

I had to wait about ten days for an appointment. This was really difficult because I didn't want to share my concern with a lot of people as I didn't want to take on anyone's fear. I mostly kept this challenge I was going through to myself, but I did speak to a select few friends who could hold with me my vision for a clear and positive outcome.

I created an affirmation to focus on while I was waiting to see the doctor again and find out what was going on. *My body and breasts are healthy. My healthy body is a reflection of my Optimal Well-Being, NOW!* The vision that I held for myself and went to again and again in my mind's eye had the doctor coming through the door to her office and saying to me,

"Everything is fine." At the end of that vision I would take a deep breath, and just let the relief wash over my body. I would stay in that place of calm, relief and gratitude. For the duration of the ten days I held this vision of a great outcome. I said the affirmation several times a day. I tried to keep myself uplifted and focused on my work with people. I trusted the Universe and God. I reached into my Optimal Well-Being toolkit and every time my mind went to a negative, I used my "Remote Control" and switched to a more positive picture. I used my breath. I always tell my clients that three deep breaths help the nervous system calm down and helps you to be grounded. I knew that worrying about the future, or dwelling on the past would not serve me well. I practiced being present, noticing my heartbeat, my surroundings, focusing on what people were saying to me rather than being in my head terrorizing myself with my thoughts. I prayed, affirmed, and visioned the outcome I desired, and worked on trusting the Universe and remembering that I was loved, supported and I still had important work to do.

When the day finally came for the re-test of my mammogram and ultrasound, I continued to breathe deeply, and moved forward in trust and surrender. While waiting for the results was far from easy, I did my best to work with my mind and tame those wild horses. As the doctor came out, I was trying to be prepared for whatever she would say. She said, "We did see something on your breast, but the good news is that it is benign." I was so relieved and happy. As I left her office I began to realize the bigger picture of why I went through this experience.

Since I was committed to spending the rest of my life supporting others to transcend their diagnosis, I felt that the Universe was having me re-experience the feelings and thoughts of what that diagnosis feels like. What I learned in this situation was that I did have the strength to face any challenge. I was prepared for the "worst case" and by being in Optimal Well-Being I knew I would be triumphant. I was fortunate, but clearly, whether it is an illness, the loss of a loved one, financial disaster, or any other "unexpected" life challenge, it is how we navigate the path of life that matters. We can't control what happens to us. We can only control how we respond.

For me, finding Optimal Well-Being and all of the techniques I used and continue to use, gives me the power to come from my highest Self with strength and the awareness that I can overcome my human limitations and step into my most powerful spiritual Self, my true essence!

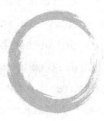

Suggested Personal Well-Being Practices

✦

When faced with an unexpected challenge,
how do you respond? Write down three positive
actions, either from this book or your own, that you
can do to support yourself.

✦

Find an affirmation that empowers you, and say it
several times throughout the day.

Final Thoughts

I sincerely hope that the ending of this book marks the beginning of your journey to Optimal Well-Being! Hopefully you can begin to see the challenge you are undergoing as a "wake-up call" to explore your authentic passions, to discover what the next chapter in your life will be, and to become the vision of your most empowered Self!

This book has given you a place to stop, and retreat from whatever challenge you are experiencing and dig a little deeper to discover the bigger picture. You have demonstrated the courage, willingness and commitment to look at that challenge as an opportunity and step away from the defining reality of your diagnosis. You have looked at your beliefs, and fears, head-on! You have connected with the deepest and most powerful part of yourself, which many people read and hear about, but may never do the experiential work to have it manifest as a reality for them.

For me, there was a purpose that was dormant in my heart until I went through my health challenge. If not for my cancer journey, Optimal Well-Being would never have awakened within me.

What may be hidden within you? What is the reason you are going through this challenge? Is there something you are supposed to do on the planet that you were not aware of? Is there something that you have been avoiding? As I have said, when we focus on something bigger than ourselves, our challenges begin to recede and the path before us becomes clear. Sharing Optimal Well-Being with the world feels like what I was born to do. What is your challenge prompting you to consider? It could be anything from sharing more love in the world and learning to love yourself, to writing that book that is in *you*, changing jobs or doing something fulfilling that makes a difference. Whatever is in your heart that your own diagnosis or challenge has led you to, now is the time to move forward in the direction of your dream. I invite you to continue with the practices of the Optimal Well-Being Path to support you to be your most powerful self and to fulfill your destiny.

There are two ways to go through any adverse circumstance. You can be a victim, and cry "poor me" to the Universe... and of course, there will be days where that is what you will do, and that is perfectly fine. But then, those are the days that can launch you to rise from the ashes like a phoenix. This is your call to awaken to your power within as co-creator, to be an inspiration and example to those that love you.

Awaken to your most powerful Self! You are here on this planet to enjoy, celebrate, and manifest the glory of who you really are! If you feel you have not come that far yet, this book is on no timeline. Learn and work with the tools in this book to manifest your goals. This is where you are on this journey, and where you take it from here is your choice. You now have the practices, space, and path to transcend your diagnosis!

My heart's desire for each and every one of you is to know you have the power to transcend all of the experiences of this life and continue your path to live your life in Optimal Well-Being.

Blessings of love and light,
Cindy Paine

Personal Well-Being Practices

Here is a quick recap of the Personal Well-Being Practices so you can review and use any specific practice when you need it.

Chapter 1: Diagnosis

✦ Write out your diagnosis story, allowing yourself to feel the feelings.

✦ Take a walk and practice feeling those feelings in your body and send them down into the earth.

✦ Experience the Grounding Meditation at http://optimalcancerjourney.com/sample-lesson/

Chapter 2: Surgery

✦ Create a vision for where you are on your diagnosis journey. Write about your desired outcome.

✦ Practice reading it before you go to sleep at night and feel the feelings of having achieved it.

Chapter 3: Post-Surgery

✦ Write about a time when you put another first at the expense of yourself.

✦ Make your list of self-loving practices you can do daily.

Chapter 4: The Plan

✦ Make a list of times you followed your intuition and it worked.

✦ Make a list of the people and places where you are not speaking up in your life.

Chapter 5: Optimal Well-Being

✦ Write out what the words "Optimal Well-Being" could mean for you?

✦ Take some time to quiet your mind: take some slow deep breaths, meditate or download a relaxation app.

Chapter 6: Physical Well-Being

✦ What would physical Optimal Well-Being be for you?

✦ List the action steps you can take to achieve physical well-being.

Chapter 7: Emotional Well-Being

✦ Discover and list what is causing stress in your life.

✦ Consider and write down the decisions you need to make to create peace and optimal emotional well-being.

Chapter 8: Mental Well-Being

✦ Create a "go to" list of positive thoughts and experiences that immerse you in good feelings.

✦ Practice using the Remote Control Technique to discipline your mind.

Chapter 9: Spiritual Well-Being

✦ Write about what gives you a feeling of connection with Spirit.

✦ Consider what you can do to support yourself in deepening that connection to Spirit.

Chapter 10: Putting It All Together

✦ Identify and write down two practices in each category to which you can commit.

✦ Begin by doing two of them this week. Continue

incorporating each practice to which you have committed into your life until they become routine.

Chapter 11: Machu Picchu

✦ Write down the specifics of what Optimal Well-Being could be for you. What are your physical, emotional, mental and spiritual goals?

✦ Pick a personal symbol that represents crossing the finish line. Make sure you really stretch beyond what you think is possible for you.

✦ Find pictures that represent you being, doing and having your goals realized.

Chapter 12: Vision

✦ Write a vision using all the parameters above.

✦ Read it each night before you go to sleep, so it marinates in your subconscious.

Chapter 13: Forgiveness

✦ Make a list of who and what you have not forgiven.

✦ Try one of the practices such as Writing a Letter and burning it; Re-Creation or Mirror Work.

Chapter 14: Trust

✦ Write about a time when you have trusted yourself, or simply trusted the process and things worked out wonderfully.

✦ Imagine if you were able to trust, what you would do with your life that you are not currently doing. Even if you're skeptical, breathe, and allow yourself to trust the process.

Chapter 15: Surrender

✦ What does Surrender mean to you?

✦ Look at a time in your life when you surrendered, when it felt like you had no control and things worked out.

Chapter 16: Telling A New Story

✦ Journal about what may be your goal or higher purpose for yourself, something you want to achieve but maybe feels out of reach.

✦ Write some action steps which will take you forward into actually achieving this Bigger Vision for yourself.

✦ Write a new story about your journey.

Chapter 17: Mining the Gifts of the Cancer Experience

✦ See if you can uncover what your "soul wound" could be. A soul wound is a behavior or pattern that you are here to heal.

✦ Make a list for yourself of the "gifts" you have received as a result of having gone through your challenging experience. These can be things you learned about yourself, blessings, and/or experiences you have had.

✦ Since "mining the gifts" may be a new practice for you, continue to look at other challenging circumstances throughout your life and seek out the treasures from them.

Chapter 18: Unexpected Challenges

✦ When faced with an unexpected challenge, how do you respond? Write down three positive actions, either from this book or your own, that you can do to support yourself.

✦ Find an affirmation that empowers you, and say it several times throughout the day.

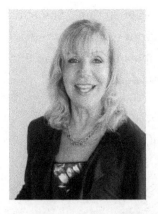

Continue the Optimal Well-Being journey with Cindy Paine by visiting her website at www.cindypaine.com and becoming a member of her community. Consider experiencing the *Optimal Well-Being in the Face of Cancer Webinar* (also found at her website) which will continue to support you on your journey with meditations and empowering visualizations.

If you are interested in further exploration of self-love or the Clear-Connect-Create Method, her book *Clear-Connect-Create: A Powerful Path to Self-Love* is available on Amazon.

Cindy Paine, a sought-after public speaker, inspires audiences with motivational messages of hope and transcendence. She leads workshops, retreats and seminars throughout the country, and has a thriving coaching business. She helps her individual clients overcome challenges, limiting beliefs and fears, providing them the keys to surpass what they believed was possible. She also assists corporate sales teams define goals and exceed expectations. She will customize a talk or retreat for your group drawing upon her experiences and the tools from her teaching to personalize the topic for your audience.

Cindy lives in West Palm Beach, Florida where she enjoys the beach, hiking, pickle-ball and helping her clients achieve greatness!